MULTIPLE SCLEROSIS

UNDERSTANDING HOW MULTIPLE SCLEROSIS OCCUR

DR. A. RAMOS

Contents

INTRODUCTION

A long-term neurological condition called multiple sclerosis (MS) affects the brain and spinal cord as well as the central nervous system (CNS). It is typified by the immune system inadvertently targeting myelin, the layer that protects nerve fibers. Numerous symptoms result from the disruption of the regular passage of electrical impulses along the neurons caused by damage to the myelin sheath.

Though its precise etiology is unknown, multiple sclerosis is classified as an autoimmune illness. It is believed to be a result of both environmental and genetic factors working together. The illness frequently manifests in the early stages of adulthood, and each person's journey is unique.

CHAPTER ONE

Important Information on Multiple Sclerosis

Damage to Myelin:

The immune system's assault on myelin causes inflammation and the development of scar tissue (sclerosis) in multiple sclerosis. This interferes with nerve cells' ability to communicate with one another, leading to a variety of neurological symptoms.

Signs:

The symptoms of multiple sclerosis (MS) can vary greatly and include weakening in the muscles, numbness or tingling, exhaustion, difficulties walking, vision problems, problems with cognition and mood, and problems with balance and coordination.

MS that Relapses but Remits (RRMS):

Relapsing-remitting MS is the most frequent type, marked by intervals of increased symptoms (relapses) interspersed with times of either partial or whole recovery (remissions).

Advance Forms:

Primary progressive MS is characterized by a slow progression of symptoms without noticeable relapses and remissions. Relapsing-remitting MS is followed by secondary progressive MS in certain people.

It can be difficult to diagnose multiple sclerosis (MS), and the process often entails a mix of clinical assessment, medical history, neurological examinations, and imaging tests like magnetic resonance imaging (MRI) to find CNS lesions.

Therapy:

MS has no known cure, but there are a number of treatments that can help control symptoms, halt the disease's development, and change how the illness develops. In order to manage multiple sclerosis, medications, physical therapy, and lifestyle changes are frequently used.

Effect on Life Quality:

An individual's quality of life may be greatly impacted by multiple sclerosis (MS), which can have an effect on relationships, work, and everyday activities. It is essential to provide supportive care and use a multidisciplinary approach incorporating medical specialists such as physical therapists, neurologists, and mental health specialists.

Studies and Conscience:

Understanding the fundamental causes of MS, enhancing diagnostic capabilities, and creating more potent treatments are the main goals of ongoing research. Raising knowledge of MS can aid in early detection, lessen stigma, and improve support for persons who are affected by the illness.

Since multiple sclerosis is a complicated and multidimensional illness, management must be approached from all angles. Improved results and a higher quality of life for MS patients are largely a result of ongoing research and a growing understanding of the disease.

Different forms of multiple sclerosis

Different clinical patterns associated with Multiple Sclerosis (MS) can result in different forms of the illness. The following are the main types of MS:

MS that Relapses but Remits (RRMS):

About 85% of people with a diagnosis of MS have RRMS, which is the most prevalent type of the disease. This kind has discrete relapses or worsenings of symptoms, interspersed with intervals of either full or partial recovery (remissions). Disease progression may be absent in between relapses.

SPMS, or secondary progressive MS:

A small percentage of people with RRMS may go on to develop secondary progressive MS. In SPMS, the disability gradually worsens over time, sometimes accompanied by relapses and remissions. Individuals may move to SPMS in different ways.

MS with Primary Progressive:

The hallmark of PPMS is a continuous increase in impairment from the beginning without noticeable relapses or remissions. Over time,

PPMS patients may see a progressive deterioration of their symptoms and incapacity. This kind makes up 10–15% of MS cases, which is less prevalent.

MS that relapses gradually (PRMS):

A less common subtype of multiple sclerosis known as PRMS is characterized by a progressive impairment from the start and sporadic superimposed relapses that may or may not lead to a partial recovery. PRMS patients might not go through distinct remission stages.

Syndrome of Clinical Isolation (CIS):

CIS is a singular episode of neurological symptoms brought on by inflammation and demyelination in the central nervous system, not a particular kind of multiple sclerosis. An individual with CIS may be diagnosed with MS if they undergo a second episode or develop new symptoms.

It's crucial to remember that the clinical course of the disease determines the MS type classification, and individual disease progression may differ. Furthermore, some people's natural course of MS has changed as a result of the introduction of disease-modifying treatments (DMTs), altering the pattern of relapses and remissions.

The variety of MS subtypes emphasizes the disease's complexity and the demand for individualized treatment plans. For MS patients to have better outcomes and a higher quality of life, early diagnosis and effective management including the use of disease-modifying medications are essential.

Reasons and Danger Elements

Although the precise etiology of multiple sclerosis (MS) is unknown, a mix of immunological, environmental, and genetic factors are thought to be involved. Here are some important things to think about in relation to the probable causes and risk factors of multiple sclerosis:

1. Immunological Components:

As an autoimmune illness, multiple sclerosis occurs when the body's own tissues are mistakenly attacked by the immune system. In multiple sclerosis (MS), inflammation and demyelination result from the immune system attacking the myelin sheath that encases nerve fibers in the central nervous system (CNS).

2. Genetic Elements:

A genetic tendency to multiple sclerosis has been demonstrated, and those who have a family history of the disease are more vulnerable. Increased vulnerability to the disease has been linked to specific genes related to immune system control and myelin formation.

3. Environmental Stressors:

While their precise functions are not entirely understood, a number of environmental factors may have a role in the development of MS.

Numerous factors have been investigated as possible causes, including geographic location (with increased occurrence in certain latitudes), exposure to specific viruses (such as Epstein-Barr virus), and vitamin D insufficiency.

4. Deficiency of Vitamin D:

Low amounts of vitamin D have been linked to a higher chance of getting multiple sclerosis (MS). Vitamin D regulates the immune system and is derived from diet and sun exposure.

5. Virus Epstein-Barr (EBV):

Epstein-Barr virus (EBV) infection has been linked to an elevated risk of multiple sclerosis (MS); however, not all cases of MS are associated with a history of EBV infection, and not all cases of EBV infection result in MS.

6. Smoking:

One modifiable risk factor for MS has been identified: smoking. Smokers may be more susceptible to the condition and may also have an impact on how the disease progresses.

7. Age and Gender:

The majority of MS patients receive their diagnosis in their twenties and thirties, with women being affected more frequently than males. But MS can strike anyone at any age, and it can also strike men and the elderly.

8. Distribution by Region:

Geographically, MS prevalence varies, with higher rates found at higher latitudes. This has given rise to the theory that vitamin D production and sunshine exposure may have an impact on the regional distribution of MS.

It's crucial to remember that many people with MS do not have any discernible risk factors, and that the presence of one or more of these risk factors does not ensure the development of MS. Understanding the genesis of multiple sclerosis involves ongoing research into the intricate interplay between genetics and environmental variables.

CHAPTER TWO

Signs and symptoms

The symptoms of multiple sclerosis (MS) can vary greatly from person to person and can take many different forms. Variations in the kind of multiple sclerosis (MS) and the afflicted parts of the central nervous system (CNS) can significantly impact the severity and duration of symptoms. The following are a few typical signs of multiple sclerosis:

Weary:

Fatigue, which can be either physical or mental and can happen even with little effort, is a common and frequently incapacitating symptom of multiple sclerosis.

Any tingling or numbness:

A common feeling among MS patients is tingling, numbness, or a "pins and needles" sensation. There are several body areas where these feelings may manifest.

Weakness of Muscles:

One common sign is weakness in the muscles, which frequently results in issues with balance and coordination. Fine motor skills and movement may be impacted by this.

Span:

Involuntary muscular spasms and rigidity are symptoms of spasticity, which makes mobility more challenging. It may be a factor in the development of muscular soreness and limited range of motion.

Issues with Vision:

Visual issues can arise from MS-related damage to the optic nerve. It is possible to experience blurred vision, diplopia (double vision), or partial or total blindness in one eye.

Issues with Coordination and Balance:

Damage to the nerves that govern these tasks can lead to irregularities in gait, impaired coordination, and problems walking.

Vertigo and dizziness:

Vertigo, a spinning or unsteady feeling, and dizziness are common symptoms in MS patients. Damage to the nerves responsible for balance and spatial orientation may be the cause of this.

Changes in cognition:

Cognitive functions can be affected by MS, which can result in issues with problem-solving, memory, attention, and information processing.

Disorders of the Bladder and Bowel:

The bladder and bowel nerves can be affected by multiple sclerosis (MS), which can result in symptoms including constipation and urine urgency, frequency, or incontinence.

Mood and Emotional Shifts:

People with Multiple Sclerosis (MS) frequently experience emotional symptoms such despair, anxiety, and mood changes. These symptoms can be impacted by the difficulties of having a chronic illness.

Suffering:

Muscle soreness, headaches, or nerve pain (neuropathic pain) can all be signs of multiple sclerosis. Pain can be persistent or sporadic.

It's crucial to remember that not everyone with MS will experience every single one of these symptoms, and that the symptoms of the disease can vary greatly. Furthermore, each person will experience the condition differently and experience the symptoms at different times. To treat MS symptoms and enhance overall quality of life, early diagnosis and thorough management including medication, rehabilitation, and supportive therapies are essential.

Identification and Medical Assessment

Multiple sclerosis (MS) diagnosis is made up of neurological exams, diagnostic tests, clinical evaluation, and medical history review. The essential components of the diagnosis and medical evaluation for MS are as follows: the procedure tries to rule out other disorders with comparable symptoms and identify the characteristic features of MS.

Clinical Assessment:

A comprehensive medical history is taken in order to evaluate the beginning, length, and course of symptoms. A person's medical history, family history, and possible exposure to environmental variables are all taken into account.

Exams Neurological:

Healthcare experts like neurologists perform neurological exams to evaluate neurological signs and symptoms such as motor function, coordination, reflexes, and sensation. Assessments of eye movements, coordination tests, and sensory checks are examples of specific assessments.

McDonald Standards:

The McDonald Criteria are commonly used clinical and imaging standards for the diagnosis of multiple sclerosis (MS). Based on clinical and imaging data, they require evidence of dispersion of lesions in time (new lesions emerging over time) and space (lesions appearing in diverse parts of the CNS).

MRIs, or magnetic resonance imaging:

The existence of distinctive lesions or plaques in the central nervous system (CNS), especially in the brain and spinal cord, can be seen by MRI, which is an essential diagnostic tool for multiple sclerosis. Active lesions may be enhanced with gadolinium contrast.

Analysis of Cerebrospinal Fluid (CSF):

A spinal tap, also known as a lumbar puncture, is a procedure used to examine the cerebrospinal fluid for indications of inflammation and the presence of particular proteins, including oligoclonal bands, which may indicate multiple sclerosis.

Potentials Aroused:

The electrical activity in the brain in reaction to stimuli, such as visual or auditory ones, is measured by evoked potential testing. Atypical reactions may suggest demyelination in particular neural circuits.

Blood Examinations:

Blood tests are used to rule out illnesses like autoimmune disorders, infections, and vitamin deficiencies that might cause similar symptoms.

Determining the Clinical Course:

Healthcare professionals identify the kind of MS, such as relapsing-remitting MS (RRMS), secondary progressive MS (SPMS), or primary progressive MS (PPMS), based on the data gathered.

Other Conditions Are Not Included:

As part of the diagnostic process, illnesses other than MS must be ruled out. It is necessary to take into account illnesses like neuromyelitis optica (NMO), acute disseminated encephalomyelitis (ADEM), and certain infections.

In order to reach a definitive diagnosis, medical professionals may combine clinical and laboratory data, as the diagnosis of MS can be complicated. Effective illness management and the initiation of suitable treatment depend on an early diagnosis. For a thorough assessment, it's critical that anyone exhibiting symptoms suggestive of multiple sclerosis seek medical attention as soon as possible.

Methods of Therapy

A multimodal strategy is used to manage multiple sclerosis (MS) with the goals of minimizing relapses, managing symptoms, and delaying the disease's development. Medication, therapy, and rehabilitation are examples of treatment approaches. Key elements of multiple sclerosis therapy techniques are as follows:

Treatments that Modify Illness (DMTs):

DMTs are drugs that alter the course of MS by lowering inflammation, decreasing the frequency and intensity of relapses, and slowing the disease's progression. There are many different types of DMTs, and the type of MS a patient has, their unique traits, and possible adverse effects are all taken into consideration while selecting a medicine.

Treatments for immune suppression:

Immunosuppressive medications may be administered to some people with more severe types of MS in order to lower inflammation and inhibit immune system function. When other DMTs are ineffective or in particular relapsing forms of MS, these drugs are frequently utilized.

Symptomatic Management:

The goal of symptomatic treatment for multiple sclerosis is to reduce individual symptoms. For instance, drugs may be recommended to address bladder dysfunction, neuropathic pain, exhaustion, and muscle rigidity.

Physical therapy and rehabilitation:

Physical therapy and rehabilitation are crucial parts of managing multiple sclerosis. Occupational therapists can assist with activities of daily living and modifications to improve function, while physical therapists can create training regimens to enhance strength, balance, and coordination.

Speech and Swallowing Therapy:

Speech therapists can help people with MS who have trouble swallowing and speaking. Exercises to enhance communication and methods to control swallowing issues are examples of therapies.

Rehabilitating Cognitive Function:

The goals of cognitive rehabilitation programs, which are frequently run by neuropsychologists, are to address cognitive deficiencies and enhance problem-solving, memory, and attention.

Changes in Diet and Lifestyle:

Overall well-being can be enhanced by leading a healthy lifestyle that includes frequent exercise, a well-balanced diet, and stress management. Certain people might gain from dietary changes, including taking supplements of vitamin D.

Handling Acute Relapses:

Acute relapses in multiple sclerosis are frequently treated with corticosteroids, such as intravenous methylprednisolone, which decrease inflammation and expedite recovery from recurrence symptoms.

Pain Control:

Patients with MS who experience pain, including neuropathic pain, may get relief from pain with drugs made especially for treating pain.

Psychological Assistance:

Managing a long-term illness such as multiple sclerosis can be difficult. Counseling and support groups are two examples of psychological care that can help people manage the emotional effects of their sickness and improve their general mental health.

Individual needs, disease features, and therapy response are taken into account while creating tailored treatment regimens. It is crucial to schedule routine check-ups with medical professionals in order to track the advancement of the condition, modify treatment regimens as necessary, and handle any new symptoms. People with multiple sclerosis have better results and a higher quality of life when they receive early diagnosis and extensive care.

Having Multiple Sclerosis

Living with multiple sclerosis (MS) means managing the obstacles that come with the disease requires a proactive and flexible approach. The following are some tactics and things to think about for people with MS:

Medical Supervision:

Seek regular consultations with medical professionals, such as neurologists and other specialists, to track the course of the condition, modify treatment regimens, and handle new symptoms. It is imperative that prescription drugs and suggested therapies be followed.

Changes in Lifestyle:

Embrace a healthy lifestyle that consists of enough sleep, a balanced diet, and frequent exercise. Sustaining an appropriate weight and engaging in physical activity are factors that can enhance general well-being.

Handling Stress:

Utilize mindfulness, meditation, relaxation techniques, or emotionally nourishing activities to manage stress. MS symptoms can be made worse by prolonged stress, so it's critical to develop practical stress-reduction techniques.

Rehabilitation and Physical Therapy:

Participate in physical therapy and rehabilitation regimens to improve your coordination, strength, flexibility, and balance. These therapies can aid with symptom management and enhance mobility in general.

Assistive technology and adaptive devices:

Examine how assistive technology and adaptive technologies can help you overcome mobility issues and make everyday tasks easier. Mobility scooters, walkers, and canes are examples of devices that can improve independence.

Mental Techniques:

Create coping mechanisms for cognitive difficulties like memory loss and concentration problems. Reminders, calendars, and organizing strategies are a few examples of useful tools.

CHAPTER THREE

Psychological Assistance:

Consult with friends, relatives, or support groups for emotional assistance. Making connections with people who comprehend the difficulties of having multiple sclerosis can offer insightful conversations, support, and a feeling of belonging.

Occupational Therapy:

Occupational therapy is a viable option for addressing difficulties associated with job and daily tasks. Occupational therapists can offer workable fixes and modifications to help jobs become more doable.

Advocacy and Education:

Keep up with developments in MS research, treatment choices, and awareness. People are more equipped to make decisions regarding their health when they are aware about the issue. In order to create awareness and foster understanding, one should also speak up for themselves and other MS patients.

Budgetary Management:

Be prepared for any monetary difficulties that may arise from having MS, such as medical costs, possible job changes, and assistance services accessibility. Stability and security can be improved with financial planning.

Frequent Inspections and Surveillance:

See your doctor on a regular basis for examinations and routine monitoring. Timely intervention is made possible by early detection of any changes or new symptoms.

Take Part in Social and Hobbit Activities:

Continue doing things that make you happy and fulfilled. Social contacts and hobbies support mental health and provide people a sense of direction in life.

Make a Future Plan:

Create long-term strategies and backup plans. Talk to loved ones about their choices for future care, and think about the financial and legal ramifications as well, such as estate planning and advance directives.

It takes a comprehensive approach to living with MS that takes care of the practical, emotional, and physical facets of life. MS patients can have happy, productive lives and feel in charge of their health by actively managing their illness, getting assistance, and adjusting to changes.

Investigations and New Treatments

The field of multiple sclerosis (MS) research is dynamic, with continuous efforts to uncover new therapeutic targets, comprehend the underlying mechanisms of the disease, and create creative treatment strategies. The following are some areas of multiple sclerosis research and new treatment developments:

Immunostimulatory Medication:

Ongoing research endeavors center on the creation of innovative immunomodulatory treatments that specifically target immune system components implicated in the inflammatory response in multiple sclerosis. This encompasses the investigation of novel medications and therapeutic approaches that alter the immune response while maintaining immune system integrity.

Neuroprotective Substances:

In an effort to preserve and guard against damage to nerve cells, researchers are looking into neuroprotective drugs. One important part of MS progression, neurodegeneration, may be slowed down or prevented by these medications.

Remyelinating Techniques:

Improving the process of myelin sheath repair, or remyelination, is a promising field of study. To encourage remyelination and possibly restore nerve function, a number of novel medications and techniques are being investigated.

Treatments with Stem Cells:

Clinical trials are investigating the safety and efficacy of stem cell therapies, such as mesenchymal stem cell (MSC) therapy and hematopoietic stem cell transplantation (HSCT), for their ability to control inflammation and reset the immune system in multiple sclerosis (MS).

Gene Treatments:

Researchers are investigating gene-editing technologies and gene-modifying tactics to target specific genes involved in immune regulation and myelin repair in an effort to change or correct genetic variables related with multiple sclerosis (MS).

Biomarkers for Tracking Illness:

Finding trustworthy biomarkers is an important part of MS research. Biomarkers can help in diagnosis, tracking the course of an illness, and forecasting how a treatment will work. Developments in the identification of biomarkers could result in more specialized and focused forms of care.

Research on Vitamin D:

Research has focused on the connection between vitamin D and multiple sclerosis. According to certain research, taking supplements of vitamin D may protect against disease or slow its course. To better understand vitamin D's involvement in MS, more research is being done.

The gut-brain axis and the microbiome:

There is ongoing research being done on the gut microbiota and its possible effects on the immune system and central nervous system. Studies are looking into how the gut-brain axis functions in multiple sclerosis and whether changing the microbiota can affect how the disease progresses.

Telemedicine and Digital Health:

In MS research, the incorporation of digital health technologies—such as wearables and telemedicine is receiving more attention. For better disease management, these technologies can increase real-time data collecting, patient involvement, and remote monitoring.

Precision Health Care:

The goal of advances in precision medicine is to customize treatment plans according to the unique characteristics of each patient, such as their genetic composition, illness subtype, and reaction to particular treatments. This strategy aims to reduce adverse effects and maximize therapeutic results.

These new treatments have the potential to completely change how MS is treated as research continues. When appropriate, people with MS are encouraged to consider taking part in research studies, as clinical trials are essential for assessing the safety and effectiveness of novel therapies. To improve our knowledge of MS and create more specialized and efficient treatments, researchers, medical professionals, and people living with the condition must continue to work together.

CONCLUSION

In conclusion, research into the complexities of multiple sclerosis (MS) and the development of new treatment options are still ongoing. MS is a neurological condition that is complex and multifaceted. As our understanding of MS has grown over time, numerous disease-modifying treatments have been created with the goal of altering the course of the illness and enhancing the lives of those who are afflicted.

New treatments that target immunomodulation, neuroprotection, and remyelination, among other areas, provide hope for more precise and potent interventions. The investigation of cutting-edge techniques like gene editing, precision medicine, and stem cell therapies demonstrates the dynamic character of MS research and the dedication to developing creative solutions.

Furthermore, the focus on holistic care which includes psychological support, symptomatic management, and rehabilitation underlines the necessity of a comprehensive strategy to address the range of issues that people with MS confront.

Collaboration between scientists, medical professionals, MS patients, advocacy organizations, and persons with MS is essential as the field of MS research continues to change. Clinical trial participation, continuous awareness campaigns, and the use of digital health technology all help to deepen our understanding of multiple sclerosis and to create more individualized and successful treatment plans.

Despite the fact that MS has no known cure, the community's combined efforts and research advancements provide hope for the disease's future. Sustaining research, early diagnosis, individualized care, and support for MS patients are critical steps on the path to better outcomes and, eventually, a society in which people with the disease can live fulfilling lives.

THE END

www.ingramcontent.com/pod-product-compliance
Lightning Source LLC
Chambersburg PA
CBHW070815280726
48660CB00015B/948